KETO FAT BOMBS

Discover 30 Easy to Follow Ketogenic Cookbook Fat Bombs recipes for Your Low-Carb Diet with Gluten-Free and wheat to Maximize your weight loss

STEPHANIE BAKER

Copyright © Stephanie Baker

All rights reserved. No part of this book may be reproduced, scanned or distributed in any printed or electronic form without permission. Please do not participate in or encourage piracy of copyrighted materials in violation of the author's rights. Purchase only authorized editions.

1
BACON EGG FAT BOMBS

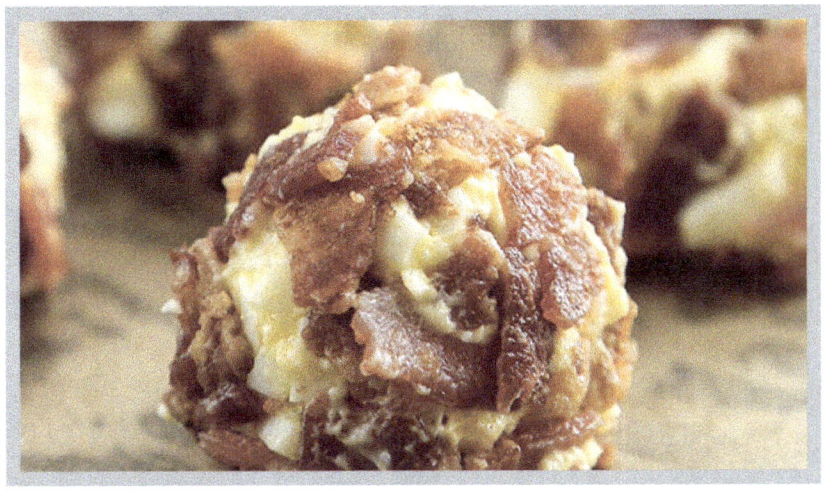

45 minutes
Portion 1

Nutritional values (per serving, 1 piece)

Net carbohydrates

0.2 grams

Protein

5 grams

Fat

18.4 grams

Calories

185 kcal

Calories from 0% carbohydrates, 11% protein, 89% fat

Total carbohydrates 0.2 g fiber 0 g sugar 0.1 g saturated fat 7.5 g sodium 297 mg (13% rda) magnesium 6 mg (1% rda) potassium 77 mg (4% emr)

INGREDIENTS (MAKES 6 FAT BOMBS)

- 2 large eggs
- 1/4 cup butter or clarified butter, softened at room temperature (55 g)
- 2 tablespoons paleo mayonnaise (30 g) (you can make your own)
- Freshly ground black pepper
- 1/4 teaspoon of sea salt or to taste
- 4 large slices of bacon (120 g)

PREPARATION

1. Preheat the oven to 190 ° c (ventilated) or 210 ° c (conventional). Line a baking sheet with parchment

paper. Lay the bacon strips on the parchment paper, leaving space, so they don't overlap. Put the pan in oven and bake for 10-15 minutes, or until golden brown. The thickness of the bacon slices determines the amount of time required. Take it out of the oven when you're done and set it aside to cool. (note: i doubled the fat bomb recipe and served them as a party snack!) Bombs of bacon and eggs

1. Get the eggs to a boil. Fill a small saucepan with water to three-quarters capacity—season with a sprinkle of salt. The eggs would not crack as a result of this. Get the water to a boil. Dip each egg in and out of the boiling water with a spoon or your hand, being careful not to burn yourself. Since the temperature change will be less dramatic, the egg will be less likely to crack. It takes about 10 minutes to boil the eggs. This timing works for large eggs. When you're done, take it off the heat and put it in a container filled with cold water. I love to love, and i always use this egg timer! After cooling, peel the mussels. Bacon egg fat bombs

1. Cut the butter into small pieces and add the peeled and quartered eggs. Blend with a fork. Bacon egg fat bombs
2. Add the mayonnaise, season with salt and pepper, and mix well. Pour in the bacon fat and mix well.

Refrigerate for 20-30 minutes or until firm, slightly greasy bombs form. Bacon egg fat bombs

1. Crumble the bacon into small pieces and prepare it for the "breading." remove the egg mixture from the refrigerator and start making six tablespoons. You can use a scoop or a scoop of ice cream. Roll each ball into bacon crumbs and arrange it on a baking sheet that will fit in the refrigerator.
2. Bacon and egg fat bombs: enjoy alone or with my latest keto bun. Eat immediately or refrigerate for up to 5 days in an airtight container.

2
GREASE THE PUMP

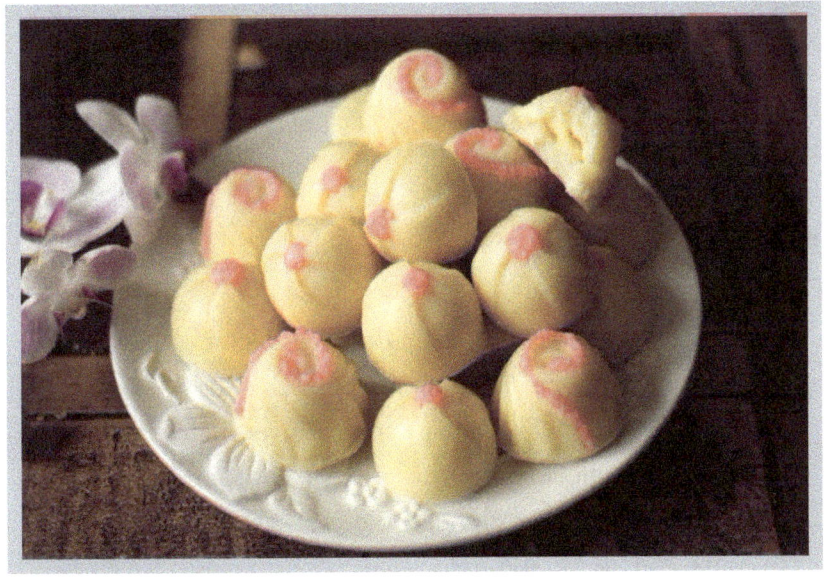

15 MINUTES
Servings: 24

. . .

INGREDIENTS

- 100 g edible cocoa butter
- ⅔ Avoid the pastry cups
- 1 teaspoon lemon extract (or another extract like cherry)
- ¼ teaspoon of Celtic sea salt

STUFFED:

1. 1 cup of Swerve (or erythritol and 1 teaspoon of stevia glycerite)
2. ½ cup lemon juice
3. 4 large eggs
4. 1 tablespoon of finely grated lemon peel
5. 8 tablespoons of coconut oil

PREPARATION

1. Place the cocoa butter in a double boiler and heat over medium heat until completely dissolved (or in a microwaveable container and heat over high heat for a minute, check and heat for 30 seconds until melted). Cocoa butter takes longer to melt than conventional fats.
2. Add a natural sweetener.
3. Mix extracts and salt.
4. Place in the truffle pan and refrigerate for about an hour until the white chocolate is firm. Or the quick

method; You can put the molds in a freezer until the end, which will only take a few minutes instead of an hour.
5. Lemon peel filling: Combine natural sweetener, lemon juice, 4 eggs and lemon peel in a medium-heavy saucepan and whisk. Add coconut oil. Beat over medium heat continuously until mixture thickens and thickly covers the back of the spoon (do not boil), about 12 minutes. Using a strainer, strain the blending into a medium cup. Consider placing the bowl in a larger bowl of ice water and whisk until the lemon curd is fully cold (about 15 minutes). It's possible to do this up to a day ahead of time.
6. MAKING THE TRUFFLE: Take the mold out of the fridge or freezer and fill it with the lemon curd filling. Then cover the filling with a layer of the cocoa butter mixture so that the lemon curd is inside and surrounded by the "white chocolate". Return to the fridge / freezer to set.
7. grades

NUTRITION COMPARISON (per serving)

Traditional fat bomb = 138 calories, 10.1 g fat, 1.1 g protein, 12 g carbohydrates

"Healthy" fat bomb = 95 calories, 10.1 g fat, 1.1 g protein, 0.2 g carbohydrates

(96% fat, 3% protein, 1% carbohydrates)

3

FUDGY CHOCOLATE MACADAMIA FAT BOMB

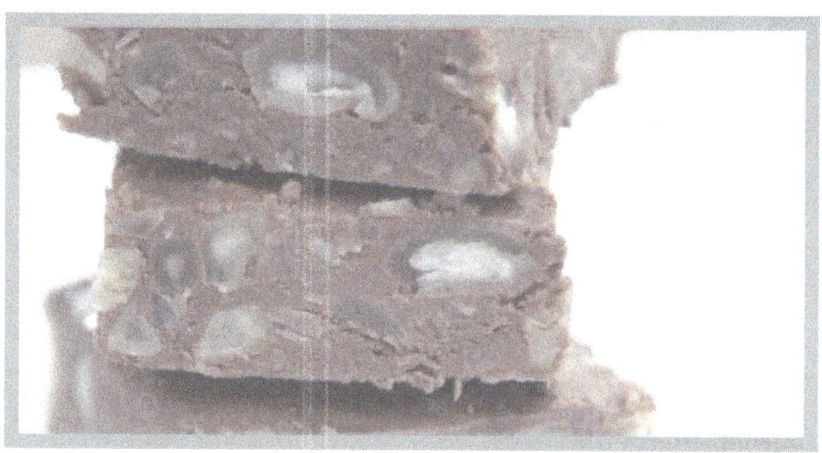

NUTRITIONAL INFORMATION
   Serving size: 6 servings
   Calories: 267
   Fats: 28gr

Carbohydrates: 3gr
Proteins: 3gr

INGREDIENTS

- 58g cocoa butter (cheaper if you make a lot of chocolate)
- 2 tablespoons of unsweetened cocoa powder
- Avoid 2 tbsp
- 112 g chopped macadamia (loose cheaper!)
- ¼ cup of cream or coconut oil for the dairy-free option

1. Manual
2. Melt the cocoa butter in a saucepan in a double boiler. (I only use another pan a little bigger, half full of water)
3. Add the cocoa powder to the saucepan.
4. Now add the spin and mix everything well until all the ingredients are well blended and dissolved.
5. Add the macadamias and mix well.
6. Return to room temperature after adding the cream and mixing thoroughly.
7. Pour the caramel into molds or cups.
8. Enable to cool before putting in the refrigerator to harden.
9. It has a much smoother consistency than chocolate and stays at room temperature.

④ PUMP RODS FOR CINNAMON SANDWICH

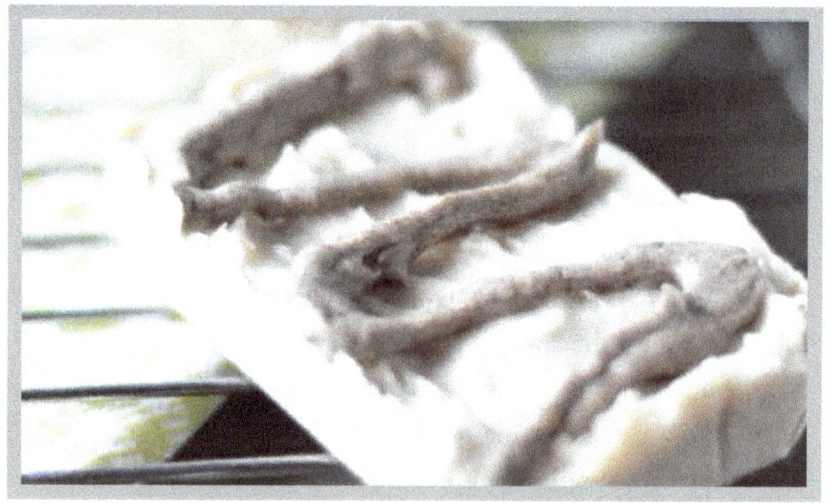

15 MINUTES

INGREDIENTS
BASE

- 1/2 cup coconut cream, cut into pieces
- 1/8 teaspoon ground cinnamon

FIRST ENAMEL

- 1 tablespoon coconut oil extra virgin (not melted)
- 1 tablespoon of almond butter or twice as much coconut oil. The bars in the photo have coconut oil frosting, but I prefer almond butter mixed with coconut oil frosting.

SECOND ENAMEL

- 1 tablespoon of coconut oil extra virgin or almond butter. I prefer almond butter
- 1/2 teaspoon ground cinnamon

PREPARATION

1. Layout a plate or mini-pan, muffin pan, etc. With the right liner (i.e., muffin liner).
2. In a bowl, mix the coconut cream and cinnamon with your hands. Pat the plate. Fill in 2 mini bread sections.
3. First frosting: In another bowl, use a whisk to mix the coconut oil and almond butter. Spread it on the coconut cream. Place the bars in the freezer for at least 5 minutes.
4. Second frosting: use a whisk to mix the frosting in a

bowl. Pour the frosting over the bars and refreeze or use.

5. I cut my rod into small pieces with a utility knife.

NUTRITIONAL INFORMATION: YIELD: 2 Serving Size: 2 servings

Amount per serving: CALORIES: 926

5
PEANUT BUTTER CHOCOLATE BALLS

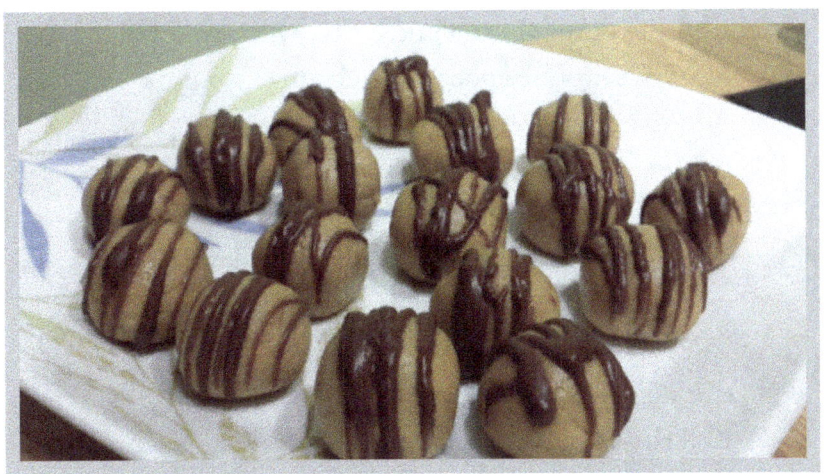

5 MINUTES

INGREDIENTS

- 1/2 cup of natural peanut butter
- 1 teaspoon of vanilla extract
- 2 tablespoons unflavored vanilla whey protein powder
- 1/2 piece of butter, softened
- 1 1/3 - 1 1/2 T of powdered sweetener (Swerve powder, xylitol powder, etc.)
- 1-2 tablespoons of coconut flour
- 1/2 cup crumbled sugar-free chocolate chips or melted sugar-free chocolate bars

PREPARATION

1. Beat the peanut butter and butter with an electric hand mixer until smooth and creamy.
2. Add the vanilla extract and protein powder to the peanut butter mixture and mix well.
3. Sprinkle the peanut butter with the powdered sweetener and mix well. The resulting dough should resemble thick sugar cookie dough. If it is too thin, add the coconut flour a teaspoon at a time until it is thick enough to form into balls.
4. Roll the dough into 30 bite-sized balls and place them in a pan lined with a non-stick coating or parchment paper.
5. Drizzle each ball with the chocolate and let the chocolate harden. For a firmer treatment, store at room temperature or in the refrigerator.
6. degrees

NUTRITION (PER BALL): 60 calories, 1.5g carbohydrates, 0.5g fiber (1 net carbohydrate), 5g fat, 3g protein

* BUCKEYES: Melt 1 1/2 cups of unsweetened chocolate with 1 tsp. Coconut oil and mix well. Freeze the peanut butter balls until firm and use a toothpick to dip them into the melted chocolate mixture. Place on a non-stick pan and rest and enjoy.

6

EASY VANILLA AND KETO FAT BOMBS

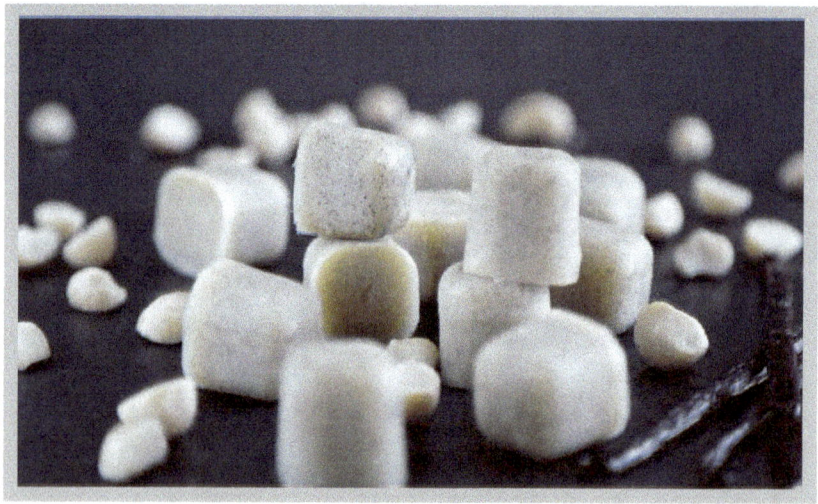

60 minutes

Nutritional values (per serving, fat bomb)

Net carbs

0.6 grams

protein

0.8 grams

Fat

14.4 grams

Calories

133 kcal

Calories from 2% carbohydrates, 2% protein, 96% fat

Total carbohydrates 1.4 g Fiber 0.8 g Sugar 0.5 g Saturated fat 6.4 g Sodium 1 mg (0% RDA) Magnesium 13 mg (3% RDA) Potassium 36 mg (2% EMR)

INGREDIENTS (MAKES 14 FAT BOMBS)

- 1 cup of unsalted macadamia nuts (130 g)
- 1/4 cup of coconut oil (55 g)
- 1/4 cup of butter or more coconut oil (55 g)
- Seeds of 1 vanilla bean or 2 teaspoons of unsweetened vanilla extract
- Optional: 10-15 drops of stevia extract.
- 2 tablespoons erythritol powder, swerve, or any other healthy low-carb sweetener from this list (20 g)

PREPARATION

1. Put the macadamia nuts in a blender and blend until smooth.
2. Easy Vanilla and Keto Fat Bombs

1. Mix with soft butter and coconut oil (at room temperature or melted in a water bath).
2. Easy Vanilla and Keto Fat Bombs

1. Add Erythritol Powder, Stevia Vanilla Extract - I love using real vanilla beans because they add fantastic flavor!
2. Easy Vanilla and Keto Fat Bombs

1. Pour into mini muffin cups or ice cube tray. You should be able to fill about 1 1/2 tablespoons of the mixture at a time for 14 servings. Refrigerate for at least 30 minutes and let it solidify.
2. Easy Vanilla and Keto Fat Bombs
3. When you're done, stay calm. Coconut oil and butter become very soft at room temperature. Simple vanilla keto fat bombs
4. Store in refrigerator up to a week.

LOW CARB BOMBS WITH HAZELNUTS AND FAT CANDIES

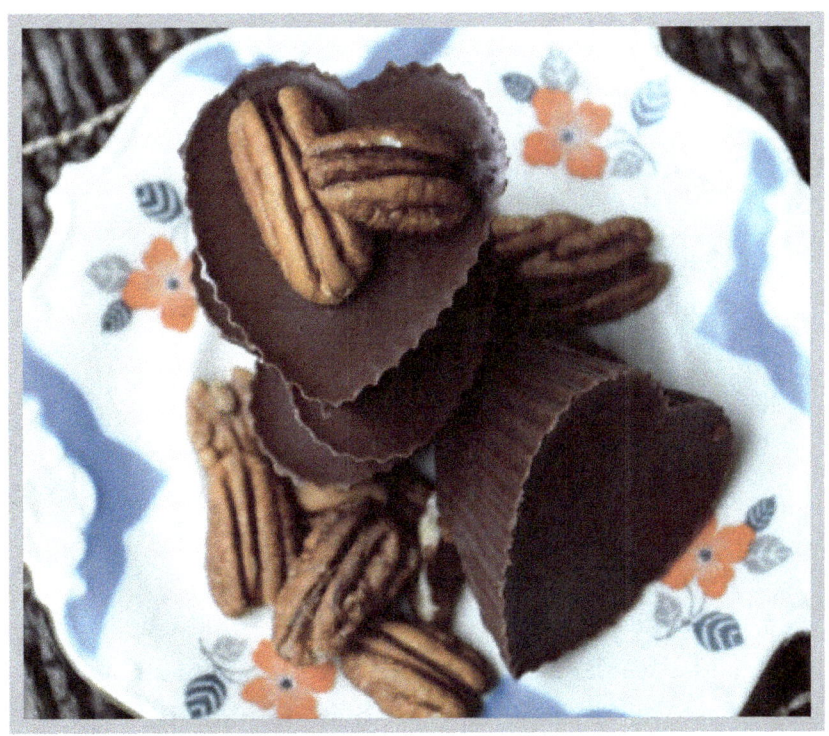

4 HOURS
Easy
Servings: 10

INGREDIENTS

- 4 oz. edible cocoa butter
- /2 cup coconut oil
- 14 tablespoons of unsweetened cocoa powder
- 4 tablespoons of erythritol (I used Swerve)
- 1/3 cup of heavy cream
- 1/2 cup walnuts, chopped
- Silicone molds

PREPARATION

1. Melt cocoa butter, coconut oil in a water bath.
2. Blend until the cocoa powder is entirely smooth.
3. Half-fill a blender with the mixture.
4. For 1-2 minutes, mix in the erythritol.
5. Mix in the milk for about 5 minutes. The sugar has dissolved in this manner.
6. Fill the silicone molds halfway with walnuts and place them on a baking sheet.
7. Pour the chocolate mixture into the desired shapes and place them in the refrigerator to cool for 4 hours.
8. Remove the shapes and have fun! * Keep refrigerated

until ready to eat; at room temperature, they can soften too much.

8
KETO SPICED COCOA COOLERS

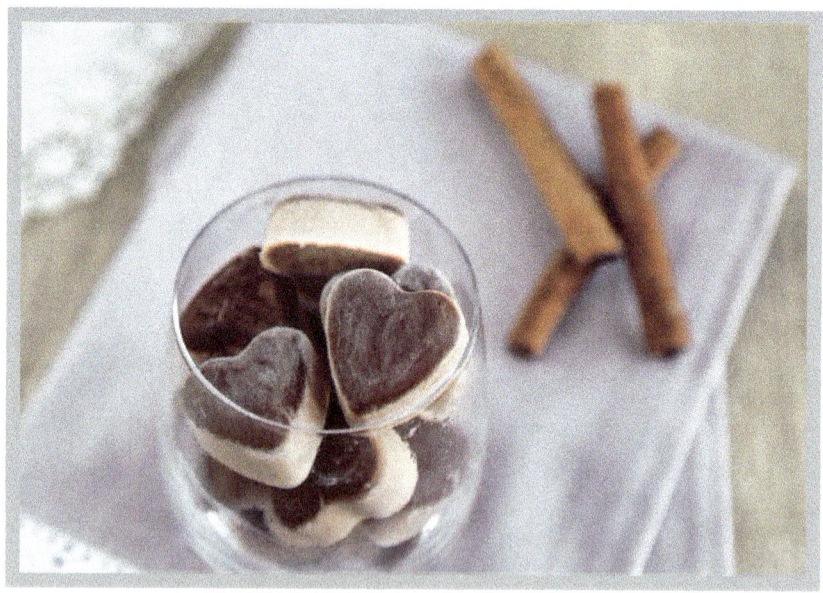

2 HOURS

Nutritional values (1 fat bomb per serving)
Net carbs

0.5 grams

protein

0.3 grams

Fat

2.5 grams

Calories

24 kcal

Calories 8% from carbohydrates, 5% from protein, 87% from fat

Total carbohydrates 0.8 g Fiber 0.3 g Sugar 0.1 g Saturated fat 2.2 g Sodium 2 mg (0% RDA) Magnesium 8 mg (2% RDA) Potassium 34 mg (2% EMR)

INGREDIENTS (MAKES ABOUT 20 FAT BOMBS)

- 1 cup cream or coconut milk; I like Aroy-D coconut milk (240ml)
- 2 tablespoons of raw cocoa powder or Dutch cocoa powder (11 g)
- 1 vanilla bean or 1 teaspoon unsweetened vanilla extract
- 1 teaspoon cinnamon
- 1/4 teaspoon cayenne pepper
- 2 tablespoons of erythritol or swerve or another healthy low-carb sweetener from this list (20 g)

OPTIONAL: 15-20 drops of liquid stevia or to taste

PREPARATION

1. All the ingredients will dissolve more quickly if you gently heat the cream or coconut milk. Keto Spiced Cocoa Coolers

1. Add all the other ingredients to the cream (or coconut milk) and mix well. Keto Spiced Cocoa Coolers

1. Place one tablespoon of liquid in each ice cube tray and place in the freezer for 1-2 hours until frozen. Coolers made with Keto Spiced Cocoa.

1. Store for up to 3 months in the freezer.

9

DARK CHOCOLATE AND RASPBERRY BOMBS

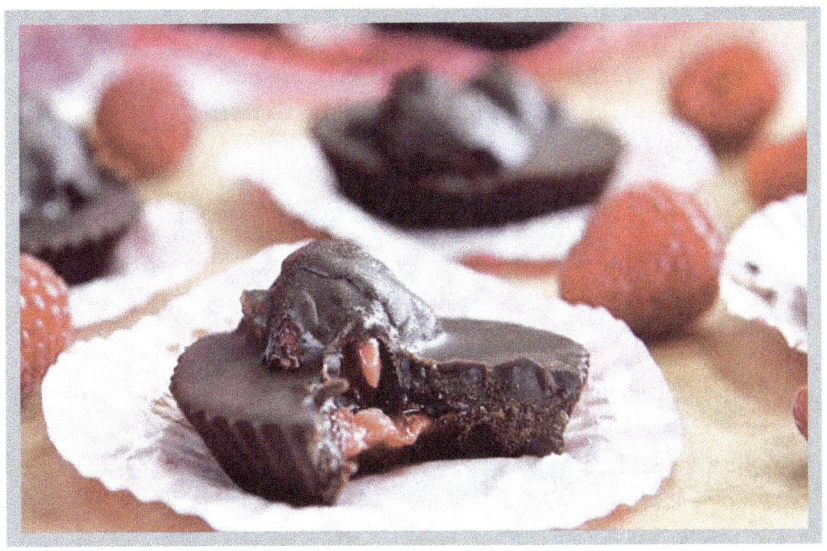

1 HR 30 min

INGREDIENTS

- 300 g dark chocolate, at least 85% cocoa
- 100 g cocoa butter
- 2 tablespoons coconut oil (30 ml)
- 1 vanilla pod or 1-2 teaspoons unsweetened vanilla extract

Optional: liquid stevia or erythritol powder to taste

ADDITIVE:

- 1 1/2 cup raspberries, fresh or frozen (180 g)
- 28 almonds (30 g)
- Artisanal chocolate:
- 1/2 cup cocoa butter (110 g)
- 3 tablespoons of coconut oil extra virgin (45 ml)
- 120 g unsweetened dark chocolate, 100% cocoa (120 g)
- 1/4 cup raw cocoa powder or Dutch-processed cocoa powder (22 g)
- 1 vanilla pod or 1 teaspoon unsweetened vanilla extract
- 1/2 cup erythritol powder or Swerve (80 g) or to taste

OPTIONAL: 20-25 drops of stevia extract or to taste

PREPARATION

1. Put the almonds in a pan and toast them for about 5

minutes to improve their taste. When you're done, transfer it to a bowl and set it aside to cool.

1. Place an almond on top of each raspberry, spread it on a baking sheet, and put it in the freezer for about an hour. You don't have to, but it will help the chocolate set faster.
2. Dark chocolate and raspberry bombs

1. Place a container over a saucepan of water and bring it to a boil. Keep it over low heat, ensure the water doesn't touch the box (or use a water bath). Put the cocoa butter, coconut oil, and unsweetened chocolate in the bowl and melt while stirring.
2. Once the chocolate mixture has melted, add the erythritol powder, bitter cocoa, stevia, and vanilla. (Note: make sure you use powdered sweetener, or the chocolate will get grainy.) Stir until well blended and set aside.
3. Place the paper muffin tins on a baking sheet and pour one tablespoon of chocolate into each one.
4. Add two frozen raspberries filled with almonds to each cup: dark chocolate and raspberry bombs.
5. Pour another spoonful of chocolate on top, making sure to cover the raspberries completely. The chocolate begins to solidify immediately—Raspberry and dark chocolate fat bombs.

6. Refrigerate for about 30 minutes or until it solidifies.
7. Dark chocolate and raspberry bombs
8. Enjoy it once it's done. Dark chocolate and raspberry bombs.
9. Store fat bombs in the refrigerator to keep them fresh in the fridge for up to 3 days. Put the remaining fat bombs in the freezer for more extended storage.

10
BULLETPROOF GREASE PUMPS

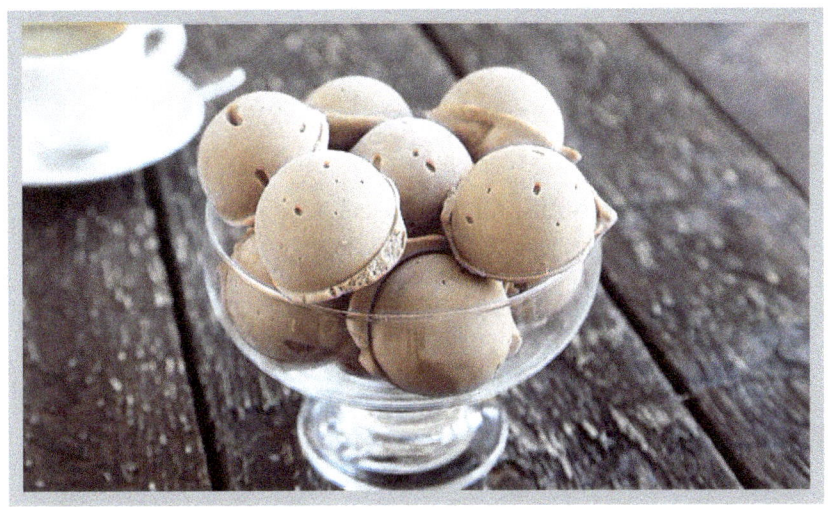

4 HOURS
   1 portion

. . .

NUTRITIONAL VALUES (1 fat bomb per serving)
Net carbs
0.4 grams
protein
0.8 grams
Fat
8.1 grams
Calories
77 kcal
Calories from 2% carbohydrates, 4% protein, 94% fat
Total carbohydrates 0.6 g Fiber 0.2 g Sugar 0.3 g Saturated fat 5.9 g Sodium 4 mg (0% RDA) Magnesium 3 mg (1% RDA) Potassium 12 mg (1% EMR)

INGREDIENTS (FOR 20 FAT BOMBS)

- 1 cup of coconut milk or mascarpone cream or whole wheat cream cheese (250 g)
- 1/4 cup of extra virgin butter or coconut oil (56 g)
- 2 tablespoons of MCT oil or brain octane oil or more coconut oil (30 ml)
- 2 tablespoons of Dutch Process cocoa powder or cocoa powder (11 g)
- 1/4 cup erythritol powder or fading (40 g)
- 10-15 drops of liquid stevia extract or to taste
- 1/2 cup of strong coffee or decaffeinated chicory (120 ml)
- Optional: 1 teaspoon unsweetened rum extract or 2-4 tablespoons dark rum

PREPARATION

1. Put the softened coconut milk cream (or mascarpone), butter or coconut oil, MCT oil and cocoa powder. Optionally, you can add Bulletproof Fat Bombs rum extract

1. Add the erythritol powder and stevia to a blender and blend until smooth. Bulletproof Grease Pumps
2. Pour in the brewed coffee (at room temperature or warm, not hot) and mix again until smooth. Pour into the refrigerator and work according to the manufacturer's instructions. Depending on the ice machine, it may take 30 to 60 minutes. Using an ice machine makes the texture smoother and creamier and also allows me to sculpt the "bomb" shapes.
3. Bulletproof Grease Pumps

1. Put about 2 tablespoons of ice in a bowl of ice. Bulletproof Grease Pumps
2. Place in the freezer for 2-3 hours or until set. Bulletproof Grease Pumps

1. Enjoy! Store in the freezer for up to 3 months.

Bulletproof Grease Pumps

LOW-CARB RECIPES FROM BUTTONI

THE PAN I used (2)
   I used a silicone ice cube tray (2)
   INGREDIENTS:

- 1 meager cup of blueberries (about 9/10 cup)

- 1 stick of butter (4 ounces)

- 3/4 cup of coconut oil

- 4 oz. cream cheese softened

- ¼ c. coconut cream

- Favorite sweetener to taste

PREPARATION

1. You can combine them in two ways: using whole berries or blending the ingredients. The latter distributes the blueberries more evenly. I like them both equally.

1. Place the silicone candy molds on a baking sheet to support and place them close to your work area. I used honeycomb silicone ice cube trays to make the ones shown above. The recipe made me 24 fat bombs of about one " x 1 ". If your molds have smaller and shallower grooves, you will get more of me.

1. Past version: In a food processor or blender, mix the berries, coconut milk, and softened cream cheese until smooth. Melt the butter and coconut oil in a saucepan over low heat. Allow cooling for 5 minutes before adding to the food processor. Puree until absolutely smooth. Sweeten with your preferred sweetener. Slowly drizzle in the sweetener, tasting and adapting to taste. I like to move the mixture to a measuring cup with a spout or a pitcher and pour it into the molds gently, not entirely. Freeze the pan for about an hour on a flat surface in the freezer. Please remove them and eat them right away, or freeze them in plastic bags.
2. Whole berry version:
3. 3-4 blueberries should be placed in each crevice of the pan.
4. Melt the butter and coconut oil in a saucepan over low heat.
5. Take off heat and set aside for 5 minutes to cool slightly.
6. Combine all remaining ingredients in a mixer or whisk, if you have one. Don't worry if the cream cheese separates a little; it will still taste nice in the finished buns.
7. Slowly drizzle in the sweetener, taste, and change the sugar to your liking.
8. Pour the mixture into the molds using a spouted pitcher or spouted measuring cup.
9. Fill in any gaps that aren't filled in.
10. Place on a flat surface in the freezer for around 1 hour.

11. Please remove them and eat them right away, or freeze them in plastic bags.

1. Whole Berry version
2. Whole Berry version

Nutritional information: The number of portions varies according to the size of the molds.

Batch 1/24: 116 calories, 13g fat, 0.44g protein, 1.02g carbohydrate, 0.18g fiber, 0.84g NET CARBOHYDRATES

VEGAN LEMON KETO FAT BOMBS

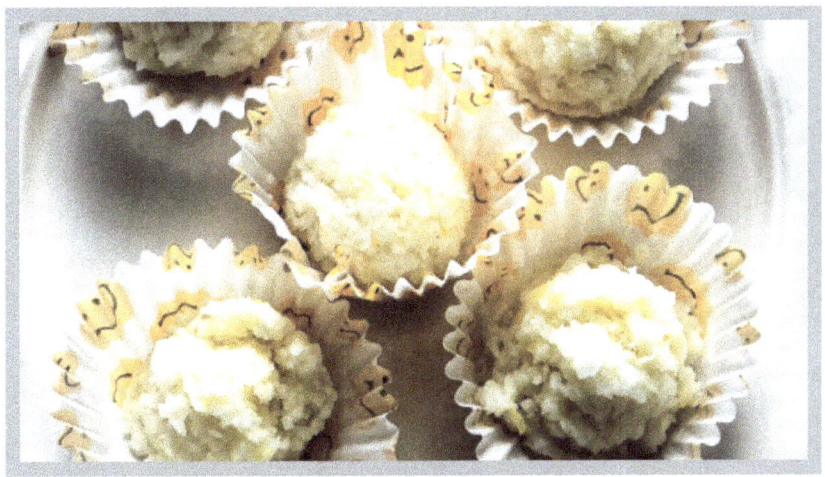

50 min
   Servings: 16

INGREDIENTS

- 1 cup dried unsweetened dry coconut
- ¼ cup coconut oil at room temperature
- 3 tablespoons erythritol sweetener powder (such as Swerve®)
- 2 tablespoons lemon zest
- 1 pinch of sea salt

PREPARATION

1. In a food processor, blend the coconut flakes for about 15 minutes or until fluffy. Mix in the coconut oil, erythritol, lemon zest, and sea salt until thoroughly combined. Fill muffin tins halfway with batter and chill for 30 minutes or until firm.

13
POPE PUMPS

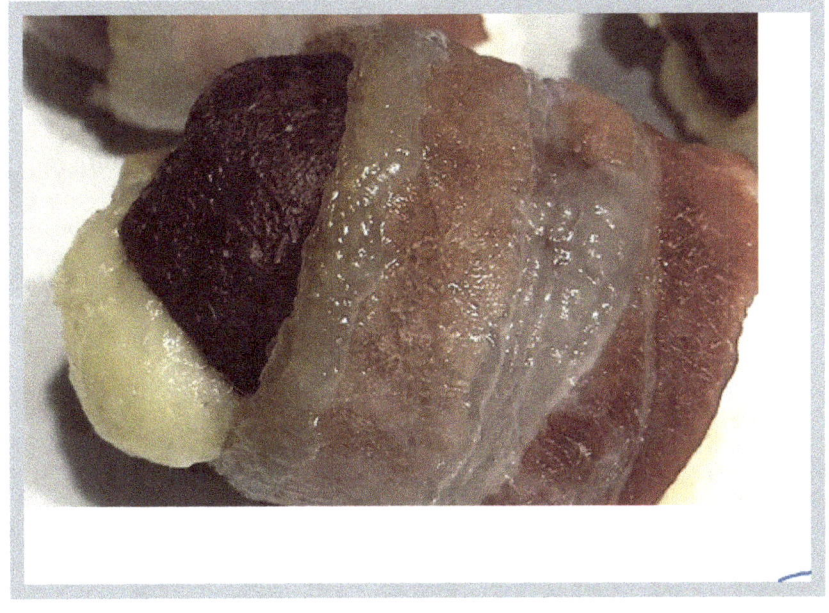

42 min
  Servings: 6

INGREDIENTS

- 2 tablespoons olive oil, divided
- 3 garlic cloves, minced
- 24 red new potatoes
- 1 cup smoked Gouda cheese
- ¼ teaspoon onion powder
- Salt and ground black pepper to taste
- ½ pound bacon, cut into thirds

PREPARATION

1. Preheat the oven to 200 ° C.
2. 1 tablespoon butter, cooked in a skillet over medium heat olive oil, cook, and stir garlic until fragrant, around 1 minute.
3. In a microwave-safe dish, position the potatoes. Mix in 1 tablespoon of olive oil thoroughly—microwave for 6 minutes, or until potatoes are tender enough to mash easily with a fork. Allow cooling before you can handle it. In a microwave-safe dish, position the potatoes. Mix in 1 tablespoon of olive oil thoroughly—microwave for 6 minutes, or until potatoes are tender enough to mash easily with a fork. Allow cooling before you can handle it.

1. Cut the potatoes in half and put the filling in a bowl. Set the potato skins aside.

1. In a bowl, mash the garlic, potato filling, Gouda cheese, onion powder, salt, and pepper. Fill the potato skins with the potato mixture and add the potato halves. Wrap a slice of bacon around each stuffed potato and place it on a baking sheet.

1. Bake in the preheated oven for 15-20 minutes until the bacon is cooked through and crisp.

NUTRITIONAL INFORMATION

Per serving: 286 calories Protein 12.5 g; Carbohydrates 25.2 g; Fat 15.4 g; Cholesterol 36.4 mg; Sodium 484 mg. Complete nutrition

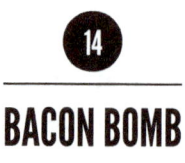

BACON BOMB

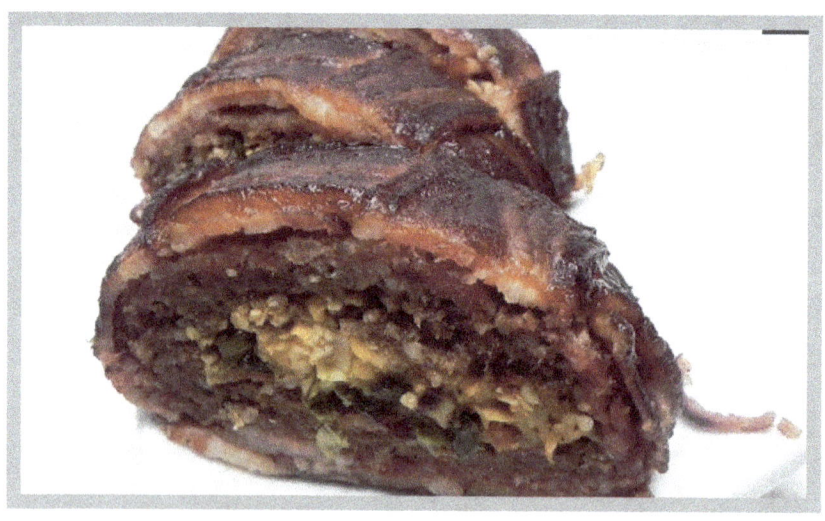

3 HOURS 40 minutes
Servings: 8

INGREDIENTS

- 2 pounds of thickly sliced bacon, divided
- 3 tablespoons of barbecue seasoning, divided or to taste
- 2 pounds of loose Italian sausage
- 1 cup of Monterey Jack cheese and finely grated cheddar cheese
- 1/4 cup diced fresh jalapeno pepper (optional)
- 2 spring onions, thinly sliced
- 4 cloves of garlic, chopped
- 1 bottle of barbecue sauce, divided
- Wood chips, soaked

PREPARATION

1. Stack and weave 1 1/2 pound slices of bacon into a 12-inch square grid. Sprinkle with one tablespoon of barbecue seasoning.

1. Place the remaining bacon in a large pan and cook over medium-high heat. Occasionally turn it for about 10 minutes until it is crispy. Cut the cooled bacon slices into pieces.

1. Place the sausage in a 1-gallon resealable plastic bag. Seal the pack most of the time; Press the link flat and

shape it into a large square. Cut off the plastic bag and throw it away. Place the sausage square on the bacon stand.

1. Scatter the pieces of bacon on the sausage square. Sprinkle with Cheddar Jack cheese, jalapenos, spring onions, and garlic. Drizzle with half of the barbecue sauce and sprinkle the remaining two tablespoons of barbecue seasoning on top.

1. Roll the sausage square into a log. Wrap the bacon rack over the sausage trunk and roll it up tightly.

1. Place the roll on a rack with the seam down. Put the grates in the smoker. Add wood chips according to the manufacturer's instructions. Smoke in the middle for about 2 hours, until it's no longer pink, then combine the roll with the rest of the barbecue sauce for the last 20 to 30 minutes. An immediately readable thermometer inserted in the center should read at least 75 °C.

1. Remove the bacon bomb from the smoker; Let it sit for 30 minutes before cutting.

1. If you want to take a crispier roll of bacon off the smoker, place it on the grill for about 5 minutes to crisp the outside, then top it with the barbecue sauce.

Nutritional information

Per serving: 609 calories; Protein 32.9 g; Carbohydrates 21.7 g; 42.6 grams of fat; Cholesterol 101.9 mg; Sodium 3440.3 mg. Complete nutrition

15

KETO CHOCOLATE PEANUT BUTTER CUPS

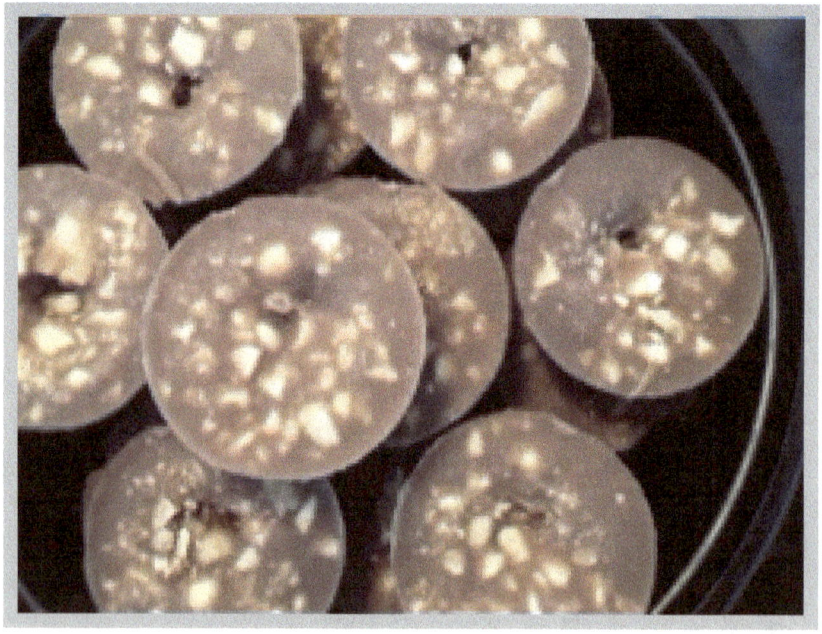

1 HOUR 18 minutes
Servings: 12th

INGREDIENTS

- 1 cup of coconut oil
- ½ cup of natural peanut butter
- 2 tablespoons of heavy cream
- 1 tablespoon cocoa powder
- 1 teaspoon of liquid stevia
- ¼ teaspoon vanilla extract
- ¼ teaspoon kosher salt
- 1 ounce chopped salted roasted peanuts

PREPARATION

1. Make saucepan over low heat, melt the coconut oil for 3-5 minutes. Blend in the peanut butter until it is entirely smooth. Combine the milk, cocoa powder, stevia liquid, vanilla extract, and salt in a mixing bowl.
2. Pour the chocolate and peanut butter mixture into 12 silicone muffin tins. Scatter the peanuts evenly over the top. Place the forms on a baking sheet.
3. Freeze the chocolate and peanut butter mixture for at least 1 hour until it solidifies. Remove the chocolate and peanut cups from the mold and put them in a plastic bag.

16
BACON AND CHEESE BOMBS

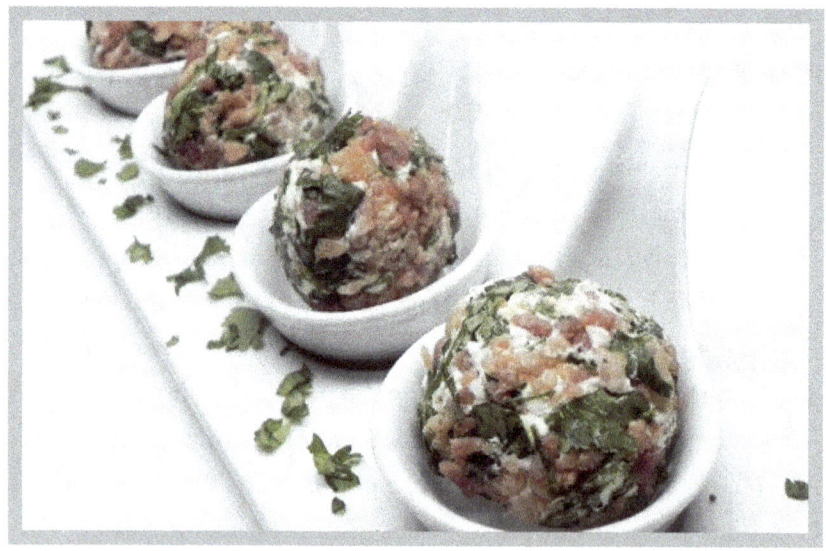

45 min
  Servings: 6

. . .

INGREDIENTS

- 4 slices of bacon
- 1 package cream cheese at room temperature
- ¼ cup of butter
- 2 tablespoons grated cheddar cheese
- ½ lime, spicy
- 1 clove garlic, minced
- 3 serrano peppers, pitted and finely chopped
- 4 sprigs of coriander, chopped

PREPARATION

1. Preheat the oven to 175 degrees Celsius. An aluminum foil can be used to line a baking sheet. Arrange the bacon strips in a sheet on top of the dough.
2. Bake in a preheated oven for about 15 minutes until golden and crisp. Drain the bacon slices on absorbent paper.
3. Combine cream cheese, butter, and cheddar cheese in a bowl. Add the lime zest, a pinch of lime juice, and garlic. Add the serrano pepper; Let cool until cool and solid, for ten mins.
4. separate chilled cream cheese mixture into six equal parts and roll into balls to form fat bombs.

1. We chop the bacon and put it in a bowl with the

coriander. Pour one fat bomb at a time into the bowl to coat them. Serve cold.

Nutritional information

Per serving: 217 calories Protein 4.1 g; Carbohydrates 1.4 g; Fat 22 g; Cholesterol 51.5 mg; Sodium 270.1 mg. Complete nutrition

GLUTEN FREE, PALEO & KETO COOKIES 'N CREAM FAT BOMBS

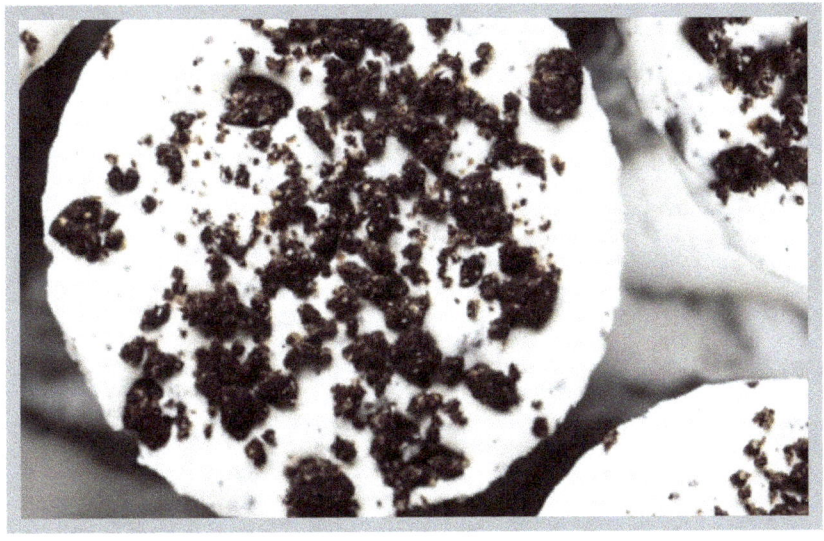

25 mins
Servings 6

. . .

INGREDIENTS

For the 'oreo cookie' crumbs

- 60 g almond flour
- 11 g cocoa powder
- 2-3 tablespoons Swerve confectioners or powdered xylitol*
- 1/2 teaspoon instant coffee optional
- pinch kosher salt
- 2 tablespoons melted grass-fed butter or ghee/coconut oil

For the vanilla cream

- 160 ml full fat coconut milk
- 2-4 tablespoons xylitol erythritol, to taste*
- pinch kosher salt
- 160 ml heavy whipping cream or chilled coconut cream (see notes)
- 2 teaspoons vanilla extract

PREPARATION

Crumbs from a 'oreo cookie'

1. In a dry skillet or pan over medium heat, lightly toast almond flour until golden and fragrant (2-4 minutes). This is vital in terms of taste, so don't miss it!

2. Toss toasted almond flour with cocoa, sweetener to taste, coffee (optional), and salt in a small mixing cup. Mix in the butter until it is fully incorporated. Around 1/3 of the mixture should be pressed into cupcake liners or silicon molds, and the remaining 2/3 should be left as 'crumbs.' When you're making the vanilla cream, put both in the freezer.

The vanilla ice cream

1. In a medium saucepan, combine the coconut milk, sweetener, and salt. Whisk until the sweetener is fully dissolved and the mixture is smooth (this should only take a few minutes). Enable to cool fully before transferring to a mixing bowl.
2. In a big chilled mixing bowl, whip heavy whipping cream or cold coconut cream until soft peaks emerge. Combine the vanilla extract, cooled coconut, and sweetener mixture in a mixing bowl. Fold in the frozen 'cookie' crumble until the mixture is smooth.

1. Fill the prepared molds with the cookies 'n cream mixture and freeze until firm. Enable 10-15 minutes for thawing before feeding.

KETO MATCHA FUDGE FAT BOMBS RECIPE

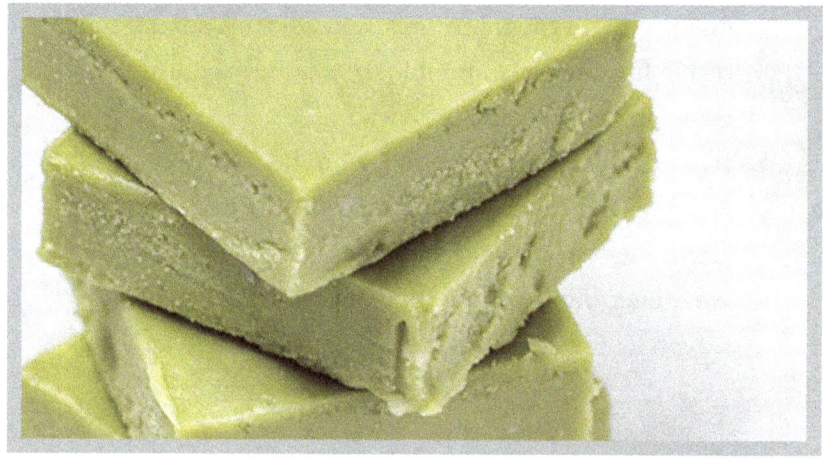

15 mins
Servings: 24

INGREDIENTS

- ounces cocoa butter
- 1/2 cup coconut butter
- 1/2 cup sugar free maple syrup
- 1/3 cup heavy cream
- 3 tablespoons coconut oil
- 2 scoops matcha mct powder
- 2 teaspoons vanilla essence

PREPARATION

1. In a small saucepan, mix all of the ingredients and cook on low heat.
2. Stir to mix all ingredients after the cocoa butter has melted.
3. Fill an 8x8 inch square cake pan with the batter and line it with parchment paper.
4. Refrigerate for at least 3 hours, or until solid.
5. Serve by cutting into 24 bits.

19
JALAPENO POPPER FAT BOMBS

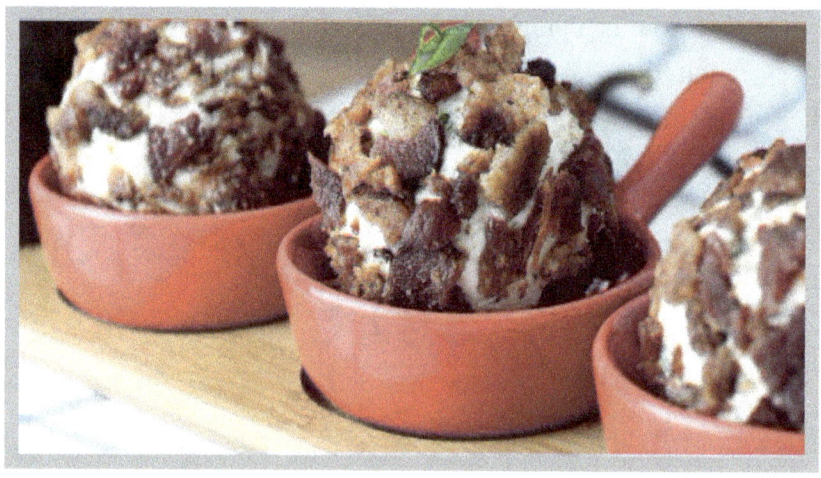

30 min
   Serving 4

INGREDIENTS

- 3 ounces cream cheese
- 3 slices bacon
- 1 medium jalapeno pepper
- ½ teaspoon dried parsley
- ¼ teaspoon onion powder
- ¼ teaspoon garlic powder
- Salt and pepper to taste

PREPARATION

1. Fry 3 bacon slices until crisp, then drain on paper towels. Bacon grease should be preserved.
2. Extract the seeds from a jalapeno pepper and dice it into small bits. Combine cream cheese, bacon fat, and spices in a mixing bowl. Season with salt and pepper to taste.
3. Place crumbled bacon on a tray. Using your hands, roll the cream cheese mixture into balls, then roll the balls in bacon.

20
LEMON FAT BOMBS

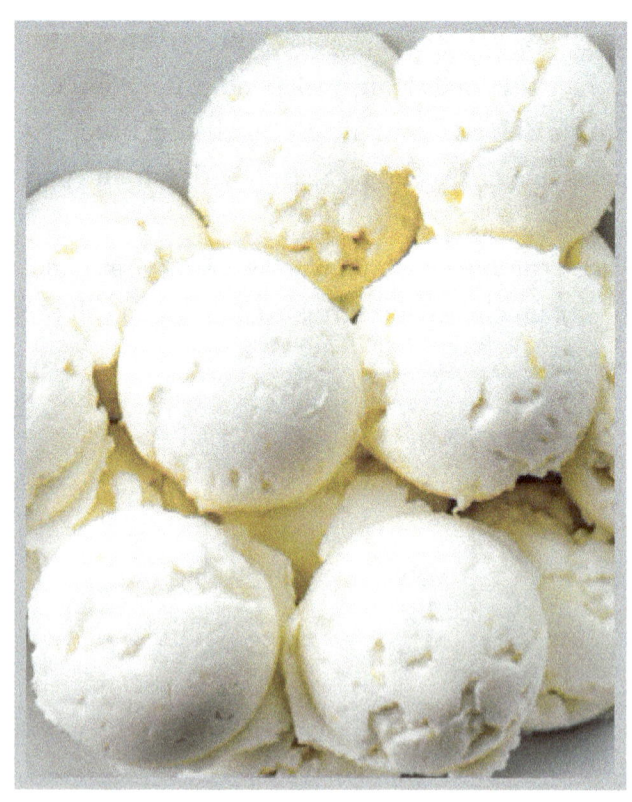

15 mins

Servings 16

INGREDIENTS

- 6 ounces cream cheese
- 4 tablespoons salted butter
- 3 tablespoons granular swerve sweetener
- 2 tablespoons lemon juice
- 1 tablespoon lemon zest

PREPARATION

1. Loosen the ingredients by allowing cream cheese and butter to stay at room temperature for 1 hour. Then, in a small cup, microwave cream cheese for around 20 seconds, or until very soft and pliable (Note 5).
2. To make the batter, whisk together the sweetener, lemon juice, and lemon zest in a large mixing bowl until thoroughly combined. Add the softened cream cheese and butter to the bowl with the lemon mixture and beat with an electric hand mixer (Note 6) until well combined and free of butter or cream cheese clumps (Note 7), scraping down the beaters and sides of the bowl as required.
3. Freeze & Serve: Divide batter evenly among round

silicone molds (Note 8) to make 16 fat bombs. Freeze for at least 2 hours before strong. Serve (Note 9) and store any leftovers in the refrigerator.

21
MAPLE PECAN FAT BOMB BARS

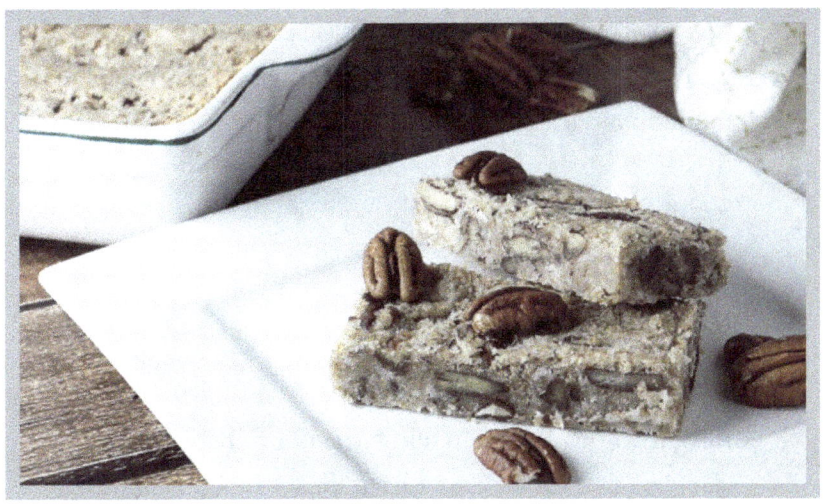

30 min
Serving 4

INGREDIENTS

- 2 cups pecan halves
- 1 cup almond flour
- ½ cup golden flaxseed meal
- ½ cup unsweetened shredded coconut
- ½ cup coconut oil
- ¼ cup "maple syrup"
- ¼ teaspoon liquid Stevia

PREPARATION

1. Preheat the oven to 350°F and toast the pecans for 6-8 minutes. Remove them from the oven and smash them with a rolling pin in a plastic container.
2. In a mixing bowl, combine all dry ingredients (including pecans).
3. Mix in the wet ingredients until a crumbly dough forms. Bake for 20-25 minutes at 350 degrees F in a casserole dish (11x7).

1. Pull from the oven and allow to cool fully before refrigerating for at least 1 hour. Serve by cutting into slices.

22

KETO PEANUT MILKBUTTER CUPS

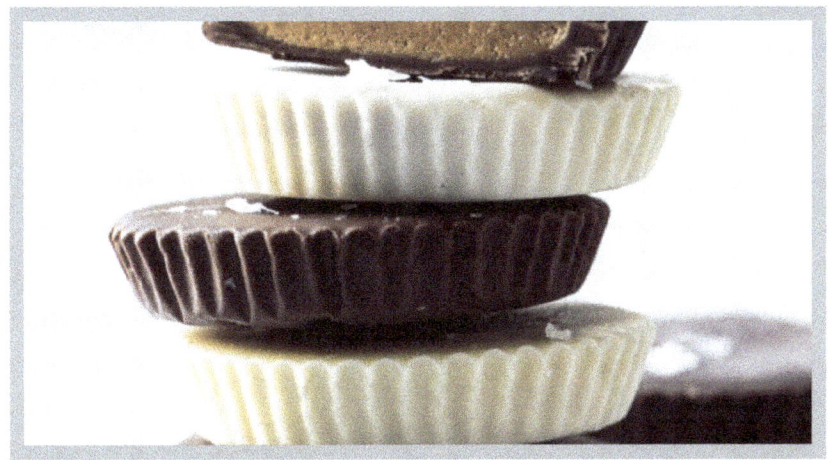

35 mins

Servings 24

INGREDIENTS

For the keto peanut butter filling

- 57 g unsalted grass-fed butter or coconut butter, at room temperature
- 14 g coconut oil or more butter*
- 1/2- 1 cup powdered allulose xylitol or erythritol, to taste (I use 1/2 cup)**
- 266 g natural peanut butter at room temperature
- 1/4-1/2 teaspoon kosher salt to taste (we use 1/2 tsp)
- For the chocolate coating
- 1 cup sugar free chocolate white, milk or dark (see notes!)
- 1-3 teaspoons coconut oil as needed
- Special equipment
- silicon molds or cupcake liners

PREPARATION

1. In a large mixing bowl, combine the butter and coconut oil (or more butter). Using an electric mixer, cream the mixture until it is completely smooth and evenly mixed. To begin, add the smallest amount of sweetener and mix until light and fluffy. Mix in the peanut butter until it is fully mixed. Check for sugar and salt, noting that the store-bought version is saltier. Delete from the equation.
2. Melt the chocolate in a water bath, stirring constantly, and change the thickness with a teaspoon of coconut oil at a time. The consistency should be pourable but thick, and the amount needed depends on the type of chocolate you're using.

3. Pour chocolate into molds and swirl it around to cover the sides (1/2-1" thick, depending on how thick you like your cups). Enable to set in the freezer for a few minutes.
4. Add a dollop of peanut butter filling, freeze for 15 minutes or until firm, then cover with a thin layer of chocolate and refrigerate until firm. Refrigerate for up to two weeks or freeze for up to three months.

23
KETO PINA COLADA FAT BOMBS

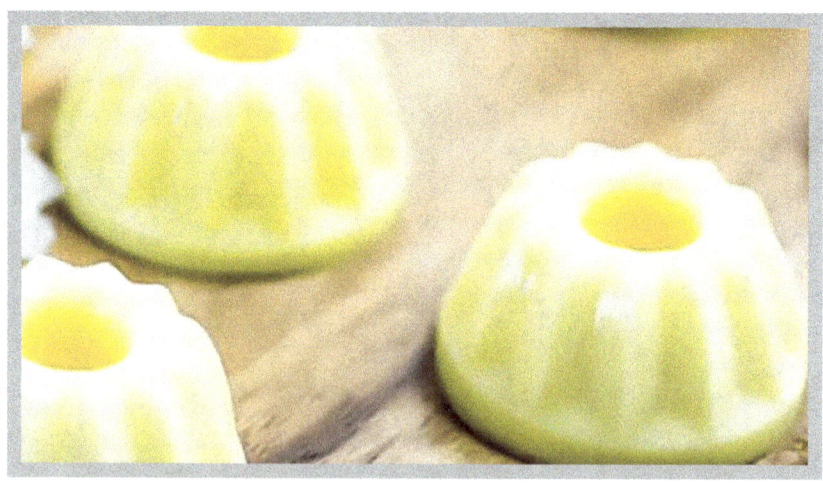

1 HR 10 mins
Servings: 16

. . .

INGREDIENTS

- 2 teaspoons pineapple essence
- 3 teaspoons Erythritol
- 2 tablespoons gelatin
- 1/2 cup boiling water
- 1/2 cup Coconut Cream
- 1 teaspoon rum extract
- 2 scoops MCT Powder [Optional]

PREPARATION

1. In a heatproof jug, dissolve the gelatin and erythritol in boiling water, then add the pineapple essence.
2. Enable 5 minutes for cooling.
3. Stir in the coconut cream and rum extract for another 2 minutes.

1. Pour into silicon molds and allow to set for at least 1 hour, depending on the size of the mold.

1. Remove the mold gently and serve. Refrigerate any leftovers.

1. [Adjustable] Add a scoop or two of MCT Powder to your fat bombs recipe if you want to spice up the taste, but make sure to thoroughly mix it in the hot water first (that may require a stick blender)

24
SAVORY PIZZA FAT BOMBS

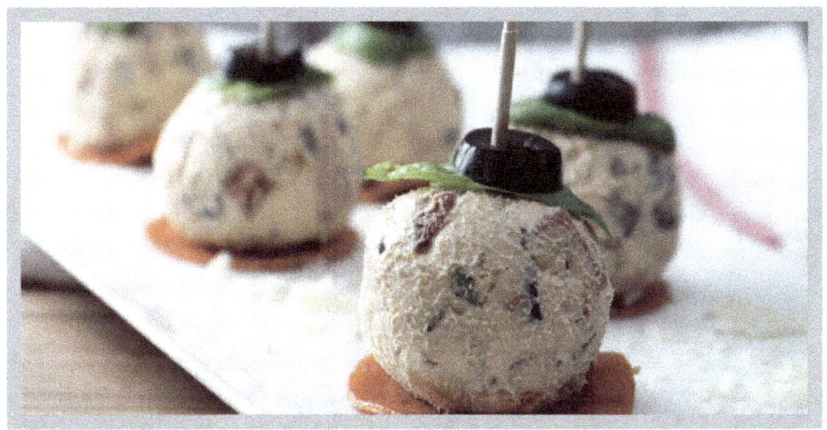

25 mins
Servings: 6

INGREDIENTS

- 4 ounces cream cheese
- 14 slices pepperoni
- 8 pitted black olives
- 2 tablespoons sun dried tomato pesto
- 2 tablespoons chopped fresh basil
- Salt and pepper to taste

PREPARATION

1. Pepperoni and olives should be sliced into small pieces.
2. Combine all of the ingredients in a mixing bowl.
3. Garnish with pepperoni, basil, and olives after forming into balls.

25

STRAWBERRY CREAM FAT BOMBS

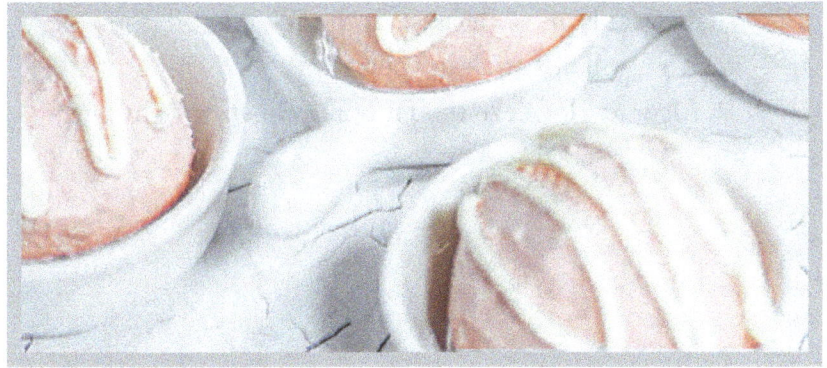

30 mins
Servings: 10

INGREDIENTS

- 6 oz Cream Cheese softened

- 5 fl.oz Double Cream
- 1 oz Vanilla Collagen Protein Powder
- 3 tbsp Coconut Oil plus extra 2 tsp for rolling
- 1 tsp Strawberry Essence

PREPARATION

1. With a hand mixer, combine all ingredients for 5 minutes, or until well mixed.
2. Refrigerate the mixture for 1 hour.
3. When the mixture has set, rub a little coconut oil into your hands and form the mixture into 10 evenly shaped fat bombs. Because of the coconut oil, the mixture will not stick to your palms.
4. Refrigerate or freeze the fat bombs in an airtight bag.

26
WHITE CHOCOLATE FAT BOMBS

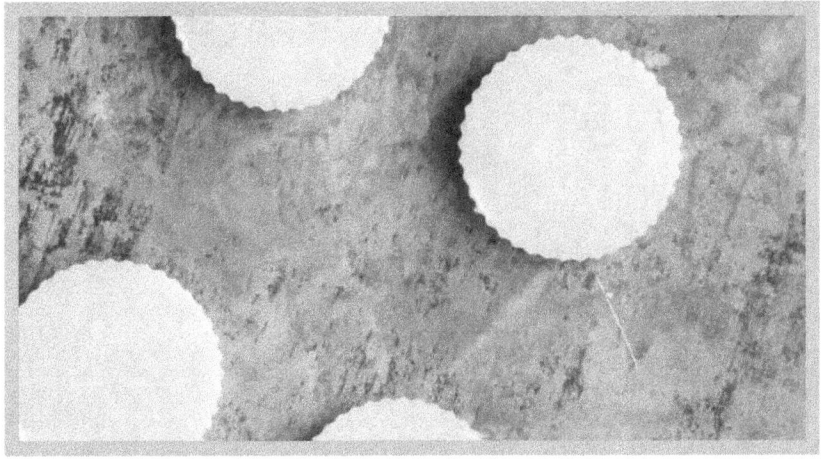

15 mins
Servings 8

INGREDIENTS

- ¼ cup cocoa butter about 25g
- ¼ cup coconut oil about 35g
- 10 drops vanilla stevia drops

PREPARATION

1. Dissolve the cocoa butter and coconut oil together in a double boiler or over low heat.
2. Take the pan from the heat and whisk in the vanilla stevia drops.
3. Pour the mixture into the molds.
4. Chill until the mixture has hardened.
5. Remove from the molds and store in the fridge.

27
KETO MILKBROWNIE BOMBS

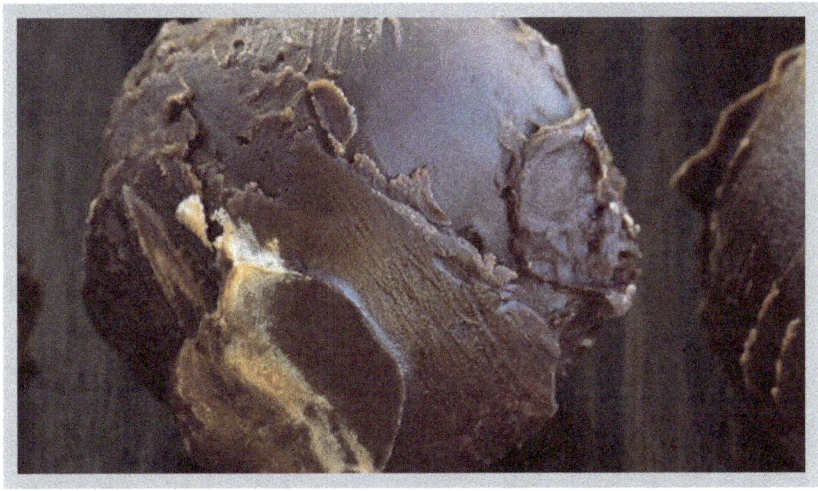

5 MINUTES
Serving 4

INGREDIENTS

- 1 cup nut butter of choice, or allergy friendly
- 2/3 cup cocoa powder
- 4-5 tbsp sweetener of choice, or as desired
- 1/4 tsp salt
- optional mini chocolate chips
- optional 2 tbsp coconut oil

PREPARATION

1. In a food processor, combine all of the ingredients and process until a smooth dough forms, scraping down the sides as required. Make balls out of the dough. Refrigerate until solid enough to scoop into balls with a mini cookie scoop if you've added melted chocolate or coconut oil. I haven't tried the recipe in a blender and am not sure whether it will fit, but please let me know if you do!

CHOCOLATE CREAM CHEESE FAT BOMBS (KETO, LOW CARB)

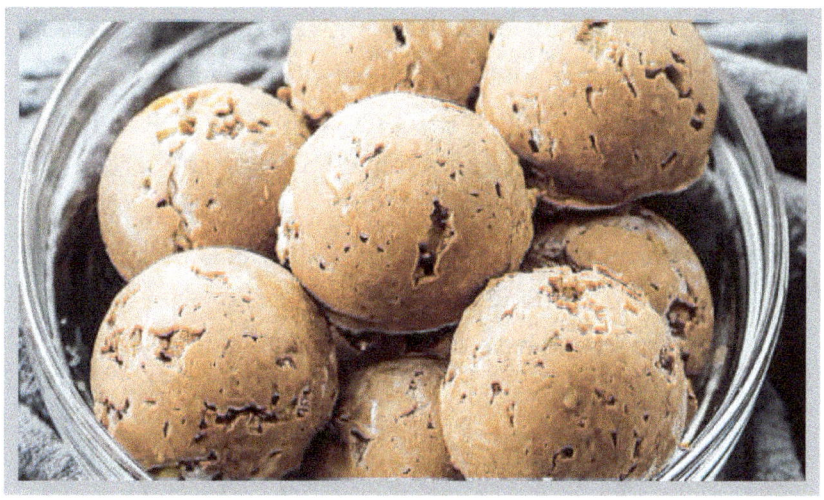

15 mins

servings 15

INGREDIENTS

- 6 ounces cream cheese
- 1/2 cup finely chopped walnuts (2 ounces weight)
- 1/3 cup chopped unsweetened baking chocolate (1.5 ounces weight)
- 3 tablespoons granular swerve sweetener (1.5 ounces weight)
- 1/2 teaspoon vanilla extract

PREPARATION

1. Allow the cream cheese to soften at room temperature before proceeding with the recipe.
2. In a heatproof cup, microwave the chopped chocolate in 20-second bursts until melted, stirring after each blast.
3. Stir in the sweetener and vanilla until all is well blended in the bowl with the melted chocolate. The mixture should have thickened to the point that it is no longer liquid.

1. Microwave the cream cheese in a separate bowl for 10 seconds, or until very soft and pliable. This is an optional move, but it makes it easier to mix the cream cheese with the other ingredients. Toss the cream cheese into the chocolate mixture in the mixing bowl.

Stir vigorously until the mixture is fully smooth. If the mixture is too thick to stir, soften it in the microwave for 5 to 10 seconds.
2. Stir in the walnuts, finely chopped, until they're uniformly dispersed.
3. Using a spatula, smooth the surface of the mixture into 15 round silicone molds. Until serving, freeze until firm, around 2 hours. Having leftovers in the freezer is a smart idea.

29
COOKIE DOUGH FAT BOMBS

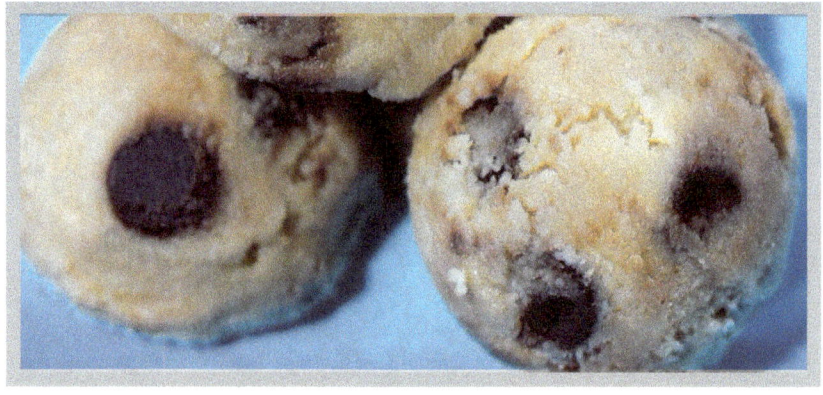

5 min
   Servings 8-10

INGREDIENTS

- 1/4 cup virgin coconut oil

- 2 tbsp sugar, or erythritol for keto
- 1/4 tsp pure vanilla extract
- scant 1/4 tsp salt
- 1 cup finely ground almond flour
- 2-4 tbsp chocolate chips, or sugar free chocolate chips

PREPARATION

Stir together all of the dry ingredients thoroughly. Stir in the wet ingredients to shape a dough. Refrigerate or freeze the balls to firm them up. Refrigerate or freeze some leftovers.

KETO BAGEL FAT BOMBS

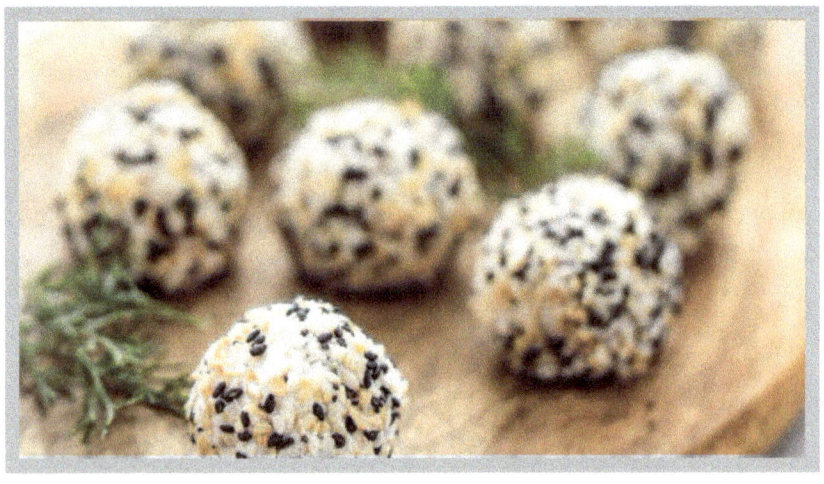

40 mins
Servings 18

. . .

INGREDIENTS

- 8 ounces Cream Cheese softened
- 2 tablespoons Chives chopped
- 1 teaspoon Dried Dill
- ¼ teaspoon White Pepper ground
- 4 ounces Smoked Salmon chopped
- Salt to taste
- ⅓ cup Everything Seasoning

PREPARATION

1. In a mixing bowl, beat the cream cheese with a hand mixer until smooth.
2. Combine the chives, dill, and pepper in a mixing dish. On medium pace, beat for 1-2 minutes, or until smooth and fluffy.
3. Mix in the smoked salmon thoroughly.

1. Taste and season with salt if necessary.

1. Measure out bite-sized balls with a cookie scoop, put them on a lined cookie sheet, and chill for 30 minutes.
2. On a tray, combine all of the seasonings.

3. Roll the fat bombs into a circular shape one at a time, then roll them in the seasoning mix. To add the seasoning to the balls, gently roll them in your hands.
4. Enjoy right away or keep refrigerated until needed.

BLACKBERRY COCONUT FAT BOMBS – PALEO

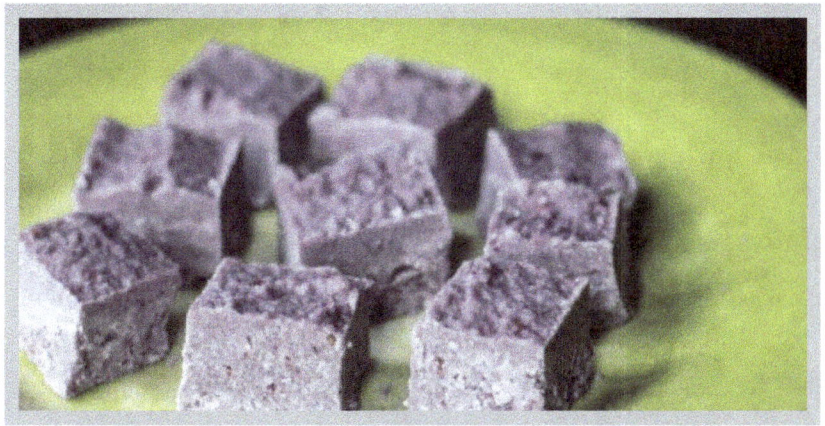

10 mins
Servings 16

INGREDIENTS

- 1 cup coconut butter
- 1 cup coconut oil
- ½ cup fresh or frozen blackberries
- ½ teaspoon SweetLeaf stevia
- ¼ teaspoon vanilla powder or ½ teaspoon vanilla extract
- 1 tablespoon lemon juice

PREPARATION

1. Heat the coconut butter, coconut oil, and frozen blackberries (if using) in a pot over medium heat until thoroughly mixed.
2. Combine the coconut oil mixture and the remaining ingredients in a food processor or handheld blender. Blend until absolutely smooth. NOTE: If the coconut oil mixture is too hot, separation will occur. There's no need to cook the berries with the coconut oil and butter if you're using fresh berries.
3. Spread into a small pan lined with parchment paper (I used a 6 6 inch container).

1. Refrigerate for at least one hour, or until the mixture has hardened.

1. Take the squares from the jar and break them into squares.

1. Refrigerate in an airtight container.

www.ingramcontent.com/pod-product-compliance
Lightning Source LLC
Chambersburg PA
CBHW062142100526
44589CB00014B/1667